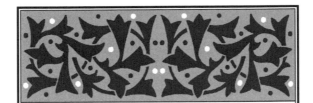

MY MILLENNIUM MEMOIR

✣

Who I Am, How I Feel,
What I Think, in the 21st Century

CHRISTINE TATE

DELACORTE PRESS

Published by
Delacorte Press
Random House, Inc.
1540 Broadway
New York, New York 10036

Delacorte Press® is a registered trademark of
Random House, Inc., and the colophon is a trademark
of Random House, Inc.

ISBN: 0-385-33431-1

Book design by Virginia Norey

Manufactured in the United States of America
Published simultaneously in Canada

August 1999

10 9 8 7 6 5 4 3 2 1

QBP

The millennium arrives, and we realize that time passes and our lives are a voyage through time. This book is designed to be a personal memoir of that voyage. A place to record your innermost thoughts about who you are, how you feel, and what you think. A place to record how you began the 21st century and to assess what was, what is, and what will be.

—Christine Tate

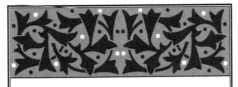

THIS BOOK
BELONGS TO

Name _____

Address

Street _____

City _____

State _____ Zip Code _____

Telephone

Home _____

Business _____

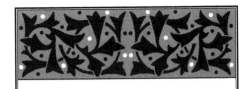

THIS IS ME

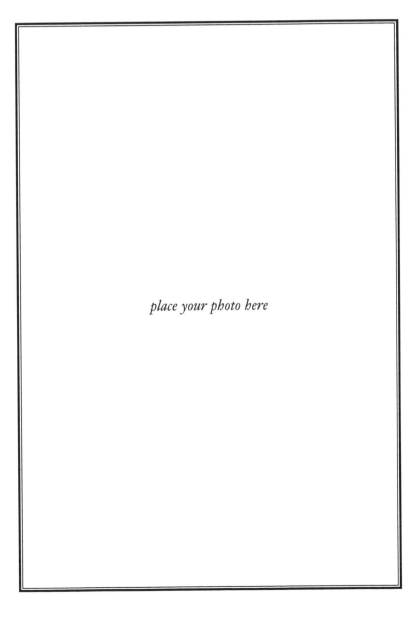

place your photo here

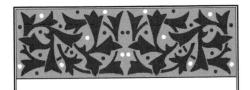

CONTENTS

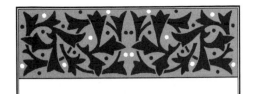

Uniquely Me

I was named after _____

My nickname is _____

I was born in _____

My birth date is (*month*) _____ (*day*) _____ (*year*) _____

A celebrity who shares my birthday is _____

My birthstone is a _____

but I'd like it to be a _____

My height is _____ but I wish it were _____

My ideal weight is _____ My current weight is _____ I'd like to weigh _____

My eye color is _____ but I wish it were _____

I ☐ wear ☐ do not wear glasses. I ☐ wear ☐ do not wear contact lenses.

My natural hair color is _____

My current hair color is _____

A way to describe my hair is ❏ straight as sticks ❏ lots of curl

    ❏ cotton candy ❏ silk ❏ straw ❏ other _____

I consider my skin _____

My nose is ❏ short ❏ long ❏ broad ❏ thin ❏ hooked ❏ pug

    ❏ cosmetically altered ❏ other _____

When I look into a mirror the feature I check out first is my _____

If I could look like anyone else it would be _____

The quality people appreciate most about me is _____

_____

The quality people like least about me is _____

_____

The languages I speak are _____

A language I would like to speak is _____

I'm most gifted at _____

My other talents are _____

_____

_____

The one talent I wish I had is _____

I   ❑ do   ❑ don't play a musical instrument—it's a _____

An instrument I'd like to learn to play is _____

My greatest achievement so far is _____

_____

What I like to do best when I'm alone is _____

_____

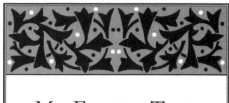

MY FAMILY TREE

My mother's name is _____

Her maiden name was _____

I call my mother ❑ Mother ❑ Mom ❑ Mama ❑ Mommy

❑ Mummy ❑ other _____

Her birth date is (*month*) _____ (*day*) _____ (*year*) _____

Her place of birth was _____

My mom's mother's name is _____

Her place of birth was _____

My mom's father's name is _____

His place of birth was _____

My mother has _____ brothers and _____ sisters.

My father's name is _____

I call my father   ❑ Father   ❑ Dad   ❑ Daddy   ❑ Pop

    ❑ Papa   ❑ other _____

His birth date is *(month)* _____ *(day)* _____ *(year)* _____

His place of birth was _____

My dad's mother's name is _____

    Her place of birth was _____

My dad's father's name is _____

    His place of birth was _____

My father has _____ brothers and _____ sisters

My parents were married on *(month)* _____ *(day)* _____ *(year)* _____

They met in the year _____ They ❑ were ❑ were not immediately drawn

    to each other. This is what happened _____

    _____

I look like my   ❑ mom   ❑ dad   ❑ other relative _____

My mom's most outstanding quality is _____

My relationship with my mom is ❑ very close ❑ warm ❑ cool ❑ cold

❑ other _____

My dad's most outstanding quality is _____

My relationship with my dad is ❑ very close ❑ warm ❑ cool ❑ cold

❑ other _____

My mother's occupation is _____

I know her dream was to be a _____

My father's occupation is _____

He always wanted to be a _____

I have _____ siblings. They are *(list names and birth dates):*

_____   _____

_____   _____

_____   _____

_____   _____

_____   _____

The TV family that most resembles my family is:

❑ the Bundys *(Married with Children)*

❑ the Huxtables *(The Cosby Show)*

❑ the Conners *(Roseanne)*

❑ the Bradys *(The Brady Bunch)*

❑ Other _____

My mother once embarrassed me by _____

_____

My reaction was _____

_____

My father once embarrassed me by _____

_____

My reaction was _____

_____

The most important thing my parents taught me was _____

_____

Something I never did in front of my parents was _____

_____

An act my parents caught me doing that I regret to this day is _____

_____

_____

I gave my parents the most joy when I _____

_____

I disappointed my folks most when I _____

_____

The relative I get along with best is _____

The one I spend the most time with is _____

My most attractive relative is _____

The relative I most confide in is _____

My marital status is _____

I have _____ children. They are *(list names and birth dates):*

_____   _____

_____   _____

_____   _____

_____   _____

_____   _____

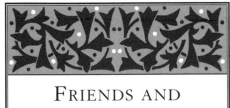

FRIENDS AND RELATIONSHIPS

The most important person in my life is _____

My best friend is _____

Other people I consider close friends are _____

_____

_____

My childhood friends were _____

_____

_____

My newest friend is _____

The person I consider a "role model" is _____

The "mentor" who taught me the most is _____

The one I look to for emotional strength is _____

The person I am most open with is _____

This one is a "fair weather" friend _____

If I were in a fix, I could call _____ at 3:00 A.M.

Someone who stuck a knife in my back is _____

how it happened _____

_____

A person I let down badly is _____

how it happened _____

_____

I should have turned the other cheek instead of causing a stir with _____

_____ because _____

_____

A friend I'd like to drop is _____

Someone I'd like to be closer to is _____

My most worthy adversary is _____

The one I most admire is _____

because _____

The people in my life in a nutshell:

The nicest _____

The smartest _____

The wisest _____

The most fun _____

The saintliest _____

The most understanding _____

The best-looking _____

The most stylish _____

The bossiest _____

The gabbiest _____

The "coolest" _____

The "squarest" _____

The most talented _____

The most difficult _____

The calmest _____

The most trustworthy _____

The least trustworthy _____

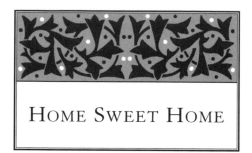

HOME SWEET HOME

I live with *(list people and pets)* _____

_____

_____

I live in a ❏ house ❏ apartment ❏ other _____

I have lived at this address since _____

Before that I lived at _____ for _____ years

My neighborhood could be described as _____

There are_____ rooms, which include_____ bedrooms and_____ baths

The other rooms are _____

_____

My monthly rent/mortgage is $_____ which I consider ❏ high ❏ fair ❏ a steal!

My other monthly expenses are *(use average):* _____

    Electricity $ _____ Gas $ _____ Telephone $ _____

    Cable TV $ _____ Other _____

_____

I would describe the decor of my home as _____

My home is *(circle your choice):*

        a. My castle

        b. Where my heart is

        c. A place to sleep

        d. A reflection of me

        e. Where I spend as little time as possible

        f. Other_____

My favorite room is _____

What I'd most like to get rid of is _____

    because _____

What I most like doing at home is _____

    and the room I do it in is _____

Household chores I enjoy are _____

Household chores I dislike are _____

At home, I can't have too many:

Mirrors	❏	Yes	❏	No
Plants/Flowers	❏	Yes	❏	No
Artwork	❏	Yes	❏	No
Books	❏	Yes	❏	No
Telephones	❏	Yes	❏	No
Videos/CDs	❏	Yes	❏	No
Electronics	❏	Yes	❏	No

Other _____

The appliance I've had for the longest time is _____

The appliance I've had to replace most is _____

My most useful kitchen gadget is _____

My most useless kitchen gadget is _____

The home improvement I'd most like to make is _____

_____

The wall colors at home are mainly _____

If I had the nerve, I'd paint my walls *(color)* _____

My preferences at home are *(circle your choice)*:

Bedroom	vs.	Dining room
Whirlpool	vs.	Swimming pool
Sofa	vs.	Easy chair
Music center	vs.	Video center
Stove	vs.	Microwave
Paintings	vs.	Photographs
Carpeting	vs.	Area rugs
Antiques	vs.	Modern
Closets	vs.	Drawers
Curtains	vs.	Shades
Wallpaper	vs.	Paint
Bookshelves	vs.	Floppy disc sleeves

I'd describe my "dream home" as _____

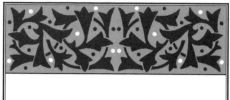

WHAT I DO

My occupation is _____

What I like about my work is _____

_____

What I don't like about my work is_____

_____

I have held this job since _____ and I expect to be there until _____

I lay my clothes out the night before	❑ Always	❑ Sometimes	❑ Rarely
I get dressed quickly	❑ Always	❑ Sometimes	❑ Rarely
I arrive at work early	❑ Always	❑ Sometimes	❑ Rarely
I stay later than I have to	❑ Always	❑ Sometimes	❑ Rarely

My confidence level at job interviews is   ❑ very high   ❑ about average   ❑ low

If I had my choice of any profession it would be _____

_____

As a child I always wanted to be a _____

My first paying job was _____

The best job I ever had was _____

     because _____

The best boss I ever had was _____

The worst job I ever had was _____

     because _____

The worst boss I ever had was _____

The reason I left my last job was _____

_____

_____

My favorite coworkers are _____

_____

The coworkers I could do without are _____

_____

I ❑ often ❑ sometimes go out with friends before going home. We usually go to _____

At work I consider myself ❑ underpaid ❑ overpaid ❑ fairly paid ❑ not paid at all

To make it through a particularly bad day, I _____

_____

I would describe my "dream job" as _____

_____

If I weren't working, this is how I'd spend my time _____

_____

_____

_____

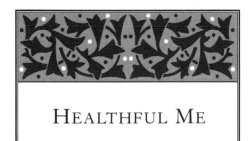

HEALTHFUL ME

I would describe my general health as _____

What I do to stay in good shape is _____
_____

Medications I take on a daily basis are _____
_____

Vitamins/minerals I take on a daily basis are _____
_____

Allergies I have are _____

My favorite form of exercise is _____

I exercise _____ times   ❑ a day   ❑ a week   ❑ a month   ❑ a year

My eating habits are   ❑ excellent   ❑ pretty good   ❑ could be better   ❑ really bad

I could improve my diet by eating more _____

I should cut down on eating _____

I should completely eliminate _____ from my diet

The "weak spot" in my body is _____

Things I do that make me feel healthy are _____

_____

Things I do to sabotage my health are _____

_____

My greatest health fear is _____

The worst illness I ever had was _____

The worst accident I ever had was _____

My "primary care" doctor is a:

    ❑ Medical doctor   ❑ Chiropractor   ❑ Knowledgeable friend

    ❑ Medical Web site   ❑ Homeopath   ❑ Relative

    ❑ Christian Science practitioner   ❑ Other _____

I visit the dentist regularly   ❏ Yes   ❏ No   My last visit was _____

If I were a physician I'd specialize in _____

In my opinion:

An apple a day keeps the doctor away	❏ True	❏ False
You are what you eat	❏ True	❏ False
Use it or lose it	❏ True	❏ False
Good health is in the genes	❏ True	❏ False
Fish is brain food	❏ True	❏ False
Carrots are good for the eyes	❏ True	❏ False
Don't swim for an hour after eating	❏ True	❏ False
Don't go to sleep with a full stomach	❏ True	❏ False
Laughter is the best medicine	❏ True	❏ False

The alternative healing methods that intrigue me are *(check all that apply):*

❏ Yoga	❏ Hypnosis	❏ Homeopathy
❏ Acupuncture	❏ Magnet therapy	❏ Herbal therapy
❏ Vitamin therapy	❏ Meditation	❏ Reflexology

❏ Other _____

The best health advice anyone ever gave me was _____

_____

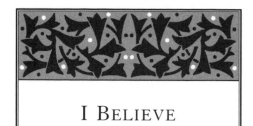

I Believe

My religious affiliation is _____

I attend services at _____ ❑ often   ❑ sometimes   ❑ never

I believe in:

      Higher power   ❑ Yes   ❑ No

      Angels   ❑ Yes   ❑ No

      Satan   ❑ Yes   ❑ No

      Good and evil   ❑ Yes   ❑ No

      Power of prayer   ❑ Yes   ❑ No

My prayers were once answered when _____

_____

I believe in heaven and hell   ❑ Yes   ❑ No   ❑ Somewhat

I envision heaven as _____

I think I was punished by a higher power when I _____

_____

As a child I believed in:

Santa Claus	❑ Yes	❑ No
The Tooth Fairy	❑ Yes	❑ No
Prayer	❑ Yes	❑ No
Miracles	❑ Yes	❑ No
Wishing wells	❑ Yes	❑ No
Witches	❑ Yes	❑ No
The Bogeyman	❑ Yes	❑ No
Ghosts	❑ Yes	❑ No

My favorite religious holiday is _____

because _____

The way I observe/celebrate this holiday is _____

_____

The literature I find most inspirational is _____

Music I find most inspirational is _____

I believe in reincarnation   ❑ Yes   ❑ No   ❑ Somewhat

In a former life I might have been _____

I'd like to come back as _____

There's always a scientific explanation   ❑ Absolutely   ❑ Maybe   ❑ No!

I consider myself a spiritual person   ❑ Absolutely   ❑ Maybe   ❑ No!

I believe in the goodness of man   ❑ Absolutely   ❑ Maybe   ❑ No!

I believe in life on other planets   ❑ Absolutely   ❑ Maybe   ❑ No!

I believe flying saucers exist   ❑ Absolutely   ❑ Maybe   ❑ No!

Vampires walk among us   ❑ Absolutely   ❑ Maybe   ❑ No!

Seeing is believing   ❑ Absolutely   ❑ Maybe   ❑ No!

I believe in luck   ❑ Yes   ❑ No   An example of "luck" I remember is _____

_____

My lucky number is _____ My good-luck piece is _____

I have been to a gambling casino   ❑ Yes   ❑ No

The games I played in a casino were _____

_____ generally   ❑ I won   ❑ I lost

My major superstitions are *(check all that apply)*:

❏ Number 13   ❏ Black cat   ❏ Walking under a ladder

❏ Spilling salt   ❏ Broken mirror   ❏ Knocking on wood

❏ Other _____

My sign of the zodiac is _____

I believe that astrology is a true science   ❏ True   ❏ False

My zodiac sign truly reflects who I am   ❏ True   ❏ False

The sign I'd really like to be is _____

The sign I'm most compatible with is _____

I check my horoscope   ❏ daily   ❏ once in a while   ❏ never

I believe in *(check all that apply)*:

❏ ESP   ❏ Card reading   ❏ Psychic reading   ❏ Crystals

❏ Palmistry   ❏ Hypnotism   ❏ Séances   ❏ Numerology

❏ Other _____

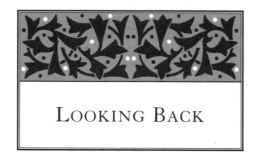

LOOKING BACK

The earliest clear memory I have is of _____

_____ and I was _____ years old.

As a child I was ❑ shy ❑ difficult ❑ hyper ❑ sickly ❑ adorable ❑ homely

❑ other _____

The best year I spent was _____ and I was _____ years old.

When I was a child, this is how we usually celebrated *(give a brief description):*

Christmas _____

_____

Thanksgiving _____

_____

Easter _____

_____

Halloween _____

_____

My birthday _____

_____

Other _____

The first valentine I received came from _____

The first valentine I sent went to _____

My early recollection of school is   ❑ yucky   ❑ I loved it   ❑ I was scared
     ❑ I can't remember a thing   ❑ other _____

My grades were usually   ❑ superior   ❑ good   ❑ average   ❑ erratic   ❑ poor

The subject I was best at was _____

My worst subject was _____

My favorite teacher was _____

I usually spent my summer vacations at _____

As a child, I was popular because _____

I was unpopular because _____

When I was a child, the one who most influenced me was _____

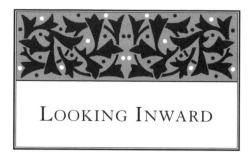

LOOKING INWARD

The things that make me happy are *(list in order of importance)*:

_____

_____

_____

Things that make me blue are *(list in order of importance):*

_____

_____

_____

The things I like most about myself are:

_____

_____

_____

The things I like least about myself are:

_____

_____

_____

My self-esteem is ❑ very high ❑ up there ❑ average ❑ LOW, low, low

If someone else takes credit for something I've done, I feel _____

_____

_____

I ignore constructive criticism	❑ Always	❑ Sometimes	❑ Never
I accept compliments graciously	❑ Always	❑ Sometimes	❑ Never
I agree with others so they'll like me	❑ Always	❑ Sometimes	❑ Never
I keep score of favors	❑ Always	❑ Sometimes	❑ Never
I have to be *very* sick to ask for help	❑ Always	❑ Sometimes	❑ Never
I have difficulty making decisions	❑ Always	❑ Sometimes	❑ Never
I am quickly angered	❑ Always	❑ Sometimes	❑ Never
I'm a perfectionist	❑ Always	❑ Sometimes	❑ Never
I collect injustices	❑ Always	❑ Sometimes	❑ Never
I'm afraid of being hurt or rejected	❑ Always	❑ Sometimes	❑ Never
I make friends easily	❑ Always	❑ Sometimes	❑ Never
I have difficulty expressing feelings	❑ Always	❑ Sometimes	❑ Never
I keep promises	❑ Always	❑ Sometimes	❑ Never
I lavish favors on those I care for	❑ Always	❑ Sometimes	❑ Never
I return phone calls promptly	❑ Always	❑ Sometimes	❑ Never

To celebrate an occasion I _____

To relieve stress I _____

To lift my spirits I often:

    Go to _____

    Listen to _____

    Speak to _____

    Read _____

    Eat _____

    Other _____

My magic formula for fun is _____

My idea of serenity is _____

I would describe myself as being *(check all that apply):*

❑ Competitive	❑ Self-assured	❑ Assertive
❑ Outgoing	❑ Submissive	❑ Shy
❑ Optimistic	❑ Pessimistic	❑ Tight
❑ Determined	❑ Moody	❑ Extravagant

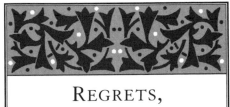

REGRETS,
I'VE HAD A FEW

A confidence I should not have revealed is _____

_____

Someone I should have told off is _____

The one I should have said "I love you" to is _____

I'm sorry I lost touch with _____

I wish I had been nicer to _____

     because _____

I regret having been nice to _____

     because _____

I broke one of the Ten Commandments when I _____

_____

I once lost my temper when _____

     and the consequences were _____

I was most affected by the death of _____

I'd have to admit that I:

Am often jealous	❏ Yes	❏ No
Avoid responsibility	❏ Yes	❏ No
Repeat secrets	❏ Yes	❏ No
Like to gossip	❏ Yes	❏ No
Harbor resentments	❏ Yes	❏ No
Can't say "No" when I mean NO!	❏ Yes	❏ No
Take credit for others' accomplishments	❏ Yes	❏ No
Tend to be verbally abusive	❏ Yes	❏ No
Blow my own horn	❏ Yes	❏ No
Harbor "could/would/should" haves	❏ Yes	❏ No
Do too many things I don't want to	❏ Yes	❏ No

A bridge I wish I hadn't burned was _____

_____

because _____

_____

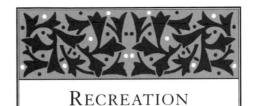

RECREATION AND LEISURE

The sport I've played most is _____

What I'm best at is _____

The one sport I wish I could play well is _____

Sports I like to attend live are _____

Sports I usually watch on TV are _____

I've ❏ attended a Super Bowl party   ❏ given one   ❏ What's a Super Bowl party?

I've been in a Super Bowl betting pool and I ❏ won ❏ lost $ _____

My favorite athlete is _____

The best role model for children is _____

The sport that should be outlawed is _____

The recreational activity I like best is _____

Outdoor activities I enjoy are *(check all that apply)*:

❏ Bicycling   ❏ Horseback riding   ❏ Motorcycling

❏ Camping   ❏ Hunting   ❏ Rafting/Canoeing

❏ Fishing   ❏ In-line skating   ❏ Snow skiing/boarding

❏ Hiking   ❏ Swimming   ❏ Snowmobiling

❏ Other _____

Indoor activities I enjoy are *(check all that apply)*:

❏ Billiards/Pool   ❏ Cooking   ❏ Entertaining

❏ Board games   ❏ Dancing   ❏ Listening to music

❏ Computer games   ❏ Darts   ❏ Watching TV/Videos

❏ Chess/Checkers   ❏ Card games   ❏ Reading

❏ Other _____

My hobbies are _____

_____

Things I like to collect are _____

_____

If money were no object, I'd collect _____

I visit museums	❏ Regularly	❏ Sometimes	❏ Rarely	❏ Never
I listen to classical music	❏ Regularly	❏ Sometimes	❏ Rarely	❏ Never
I listen to pop music	❏ Regularly	❏ Sometimes	❏ Rarely	❏ Never
I attend the ballet	❏ Regularly	❏ Sometimes	❏ Rarely	❏ Never
I attend plays	❏ Regularly	❏ Sometimes	❏ Rarely	❏ Never
I attend rock concerts	❏ Regularly	❏ Sometimes	❏ Rarely	❏ Never
I go to the opera	❏ Regularly	❏ Sometimes	❏ Rarely	❏ Never
I go out dancing	❏ Regularly	❏ Sometimes	❏ Rarely	❏ Never
I read books	❏ Regularly	❏ Sometimes	❏ Rarely	❏ Never

My favorite book of all time is _____

My favorite kinds of books include (check off all that apply):

❏ Mystery   ❏ Biography   ❏ Romance   ❏ Adventure

❏ Historical   ❏ How-to   ❏ Cookbooks   ❏ Spiritual

❏ Self-improvement   ❏ Other _____

_____

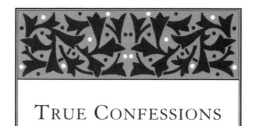

TRUE CONFESSIONS

Things I do on a regular basis:

Pay compliments   ❏ Yes   ❏ No

Make someone happy   ❏ Yes   ❏ No

Make someone unhappy   ❏ Yes   ❏ No

Make friends   ❏ Yes   ❏ No

Carry grudges   ❏ Yes   ❏ No

Forgive and forget   ❏ Yes   ❏ No

Stretch the truth   ❏ Yes   ❏ No

Count my blessings   ❏ Yes   ❏ No

Support a charity   ❏ Yes   ❏ No

Smile   ❏ Yes   ❏ No

Cry   ❏ Yes   ❏ No

Worry   ❏ Yes   ❏ No

Other _____

_____

What I do too much of is:

Smoke	❏ Yes	❏ No
Drink	❏ Yes	❏ No
Curse	❏ Yes	❏ No
Exercise	❏ Yes	❏ No
Nag	❏ Yes	❏ No
Surf the Web	❏ Yes	❏ No
Work	❏ Yes	❏ No
Eat	❏ Yes	❏ No
Fantasize	❏ Yes	❏ No
Analyze	❏ Yes	❏ No
Talk	❏ Yes	❏ No
Isolate myself	❏ Yes	❏ No
Shop	❏ Yes	❏ No
Think	❏ Yes	❏ No
Argue	❏ Yes	❏ No
Apologize	❏ Yes	❏ No
Sleep	❏ Yes	❏ No
Judge others	❏ Yes	❏ No
Compete	❏ Yes	❏ No
Procrastinate	❏ Yes	❏ No
Spend money	❏ Yes	❏ No

Other _____

A celebrity I could be obsessed with is _____

Things that frighten me are _____

_____

_____

_____

The sins I most identify with are *(check those that apply):*

    ❑ Anger

    ❑ Greed

    ❑ Sloth

    ❑ Envy

    ❑ Pride

    ❑ Lust

    ❑ Gluttony

The one luxury I can't have enough of is _____

_____

What excites me the most is _____

_____

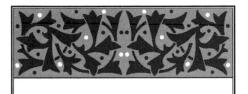

YES, I CAN!

I know how to:

Knit	❏ Well	❏ Somewhat	❏ Poorly	❏ Not at all
Paint a room	❏ Well	❏ Somewhat	❏ Poorly	❏ Not at all
Swing a golf club	❏ Well	❏ Somewhat	❏ Poorly	❏ Not at all
Ride a bike	❏ Well	❏ Somewhat	❏ Poorly	❏ Not at all
Sew	❏ Well	❏ Somewhat	❏ Poorly	❏ Not at all
Play tennis	❏ Well	❏ Somewhat	❏ Poorly	❏ Not at all
Dance the tango	❏ Well	❏ Somewhat	❏ Poorly	❏ Not at all
Bake a cake	❏ Well	❏ Somewhat	❏ Poorly	❏ Not at all
Use a computer	❏ Well	❏ Somewhat	❏ Poorly	❏ Not at all
Drive	❏ Well	❏ Somewhat	❏ Poorly	❏ Not at all
Change a tire	❏ Well	❏ Somewhat	❏ Poorly	❏ Not at all
Ice skate	❏ Well	❏ Somewhat	❏ Poorly	❏ Not at all
Change a diaper	❏ Well	❏ Somewhat	❏ Poorly	❏ Not at all
Cook	❏ Well	❏ Somewhat	❏ Poorly	❏ Not at all
Use a video camera	❏ Well	❏ Somewhat	❏ Poorly	❏ Not at all

Sing	❏ Well	❏ Somewhat	❏ Poorly	❏ Not at all
Give a manicure	❏ Well	❏ Somewhat	❏ Poorly	❏ Not at all
Program a VCR	❏ Well	❏ Somewhat	❏ Poorly	❏ Not at all
Train a dog	❏ Well	❏ Somewhat	❏ Poorly	❏ Not at all
Play piano	❏ Well	❏ Somewhat	❏ Poorly	❏ Not at all
Prepare a fire	❏ Well	❏ Somewhat	❏ Poorly	❏ Not at all
Play bridge	❏ Well	❏ Somewhat	❏ Poorly	❏ Not at all
Play chess	❏ Well	❏ Somewhat	❏ Poorly	❏ Not at all
Play poker	❏ Well	❏ Somewhat	❏ Poorly	❏ Not at all
Raise houseplants	❏ Well	❏ Somewhat	❏ Poorly	❏ Not at all
Arrange flowers	❏ Well	❏ Somewhat	❏ Poorly	❏ Not at all
Give a large party	❏ Well	❏ Somewhat	❏ Poorly	❏ Not at all
Read a road map	❏ Well	❏ Somewhat	❏ Poorly	❏ Not at all
Make minor repairs	❏ Well	❏ Somewhat	❏ Poorly	❏ Not at all
Swim	❏ Well	❏ Somewhat	❏ Poorly	❏ Not at all
Dive	❏ Well	❏ Somewhat	❏ Poorly	❏ Not at all
Balance a checkbook	❏ Well	❏ Somewhat	❏ Poorly	❏ Not at all

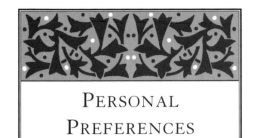

PERSONAL PREFERENCES

The best place to watch a sunset is _____

My favorite color is _____

Of the four seasons, the one I wish would last longer is _____

     because _____

The flower I prefer is _____

My favorite houseplant is _____

The tree I like most is _____

My favorite term of endearment is _____

My favorite aromas *(fill in your favorites):*

     Food _____

     Herb/Spice _____

     Flower _____

     Perfume _____

     Other _____

My favorite vacation spot is _____

The car type I prefer is ❏ sedan ❏ coupe ❏ convertible ❏ other _____

The style of painting I like best is _____

My favorite place for a long walk is _____

My favorite places to browse are *(check all that apply):*

    ❏ Antique stores   ❏ Hardware stores   ❏ The mall

    ❏ Toy shops   ❏ Department stores   ❏ Boutiques

    ❏ The Web   ❏ Bookstores

    ❏ Other _____

My favorite *(fill in your favorites):*

    Gemstone _____

    Brand of watch _____

    Fruit _____

    Boy's name _____

    Girl's name _____

    Day of the year _____

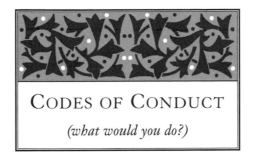

CODES OF CONDUCT

(what would you do?)

I find my friend's spouse is cheating. I _____

_____

The bank ATM gives me too much money. I _____

_____

I open a gift I know is "recycled." I say _____

_____

A superior credits me for someone else's project. I _____

_____

A coworker asks if I like her dress, which is awful. I say _____

_____

My neighbor's child has no ear for music. After her recital, I say _____

_____

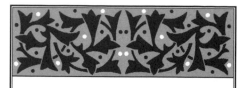

A WALK ON
THE WILD SIDE

	I might	I'd prefer root canal
Give all my money to charity	_____	_____
Take my phone off the hook for a week	_____	_____
Change my hair color	_____	_____
Take up skydiving	_____	_____
Give/take back the engagement ring	_____	_____
Study to be an opera singer	_____	_____
Ride a bike through a tough neighborhood	_____	_____
Change my first name	_____	_____
Eat lobster on a first date	_____	_____
Convert to another religion	_____	_____
Go bear hunting	_____	_____
Cross-dress while food shopping	_____	_____
Stiff the waiter for bad service	_____	_____
Go white-water rafting	_____	_____
Eat monkey stew	_____	_____
Learn to fly a plane	_____	_____
Have plastic surgery	_____	_____
Go into politics	_____	_____
Become a vegetarian	_____	_____

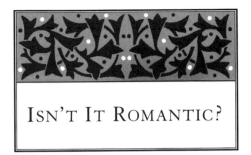

Isn't It Romantic?

Meaningful "firsts" in my life *(list with whom and your age):*

Crush _____ Age _____

Date _____ Age _____

Kiss _____ Age _____

Steady _____ Age _____

Love _____ Age _____

The most romantic thing that happened to me was _____

_____

The most romantic thing I ever did for anyone was _____

_____

The most romantic song I ever heard was _____

I'm most drawn to a person's beautiful ❑ eyes ❑ smile

The least important physical feature is _____

In my opinion:

A man must be masculine	❏ True	❏ False
A woman should be feminine	❏ True	❏ False
Opposites attract	❏ True	❏ False
Out of sight, out of mind	❏ True	❏ False
Absence makes the heart grow fonder	❏ True	❏ False

The number of times I have been in love is _____

I could flirt forever with _____

A relationship should be   ❏ 50–50   ❏ played by ear   ❏ all or nothing

What I look for in that "special someone" is *(rate 10 = most important to 1 = least important)*:

____ Looks	____ Intelligence	____ Culture
____ Money	____ Honesty	____ Professional success
____ Power	____ Confidence	____ Kindness
____ Personality	____ Integrity	____ Assertiveness
____ Humor	____ Style	____ Tact
____ Spirituality	____ Imagination	____ Sexiness

A past romance I cherish is _____ _____

Someone who broke my heart was _____

The one whose heart I broke was _____

The one that got away was _____

The one of my dreams knows how to:

Dance	❏ Important	❏ I couldn't care less
Make money	❏ Important	❏ I couldn't care less
Have fun	❏ Important	❏ I couldn't care less
Dress with style	❏ Important	❏ I couldn't care less
Be a good parent	❏ Important	❏ I couldn't care less
Be diplomatic	❏ Important	❏ I couldn't care less
Make me feel special	❏ Important	❏ I couldn't care less
Make me feel needed	❏ Important	❏ I couldn't care less
Kiss and make up	❏ Important	❏ I couldn't care less
Be faithful	❏ Important	❏ I couldn't care less
Appreciate music	❏ Important	❏ I couldn't care less
Love animals	❏ Important	❏ I couldn't care less

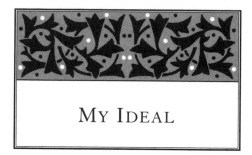

My Ideal

The love of my life would have the *(fill in the name of a celebrity/famous person):*

Looks of _____

Personality of _____

Body of _____

Brains of _____

Eyes of _____

Hair of _____

Smile of _____

Talent of _____

Wealth of _____

Power of _____

Humor of _____

Tenderness of _____

Generosity of _____

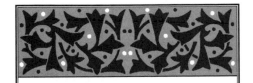

TAKING SIDES

(circle your choice)

Bagels	vs.	Muffins
Blonde	vs.	Brunette
Teletubbies	vs.	Barney
Rap	vs.	Metal
E-mail	vs.	Snail mail
Slapstick	vs.	Wit
Cowboys	vs.	Indians
Beach	vs.	Mountains
Rolls	vs.	Mercedes
Solitude	vs.	Crowds
Michael Jordan	vs.	Mark McGwire
Salsa	vs.	Ketchup
Active	vs.	Reactive
Driving	vs.	Driven
Emeralds	vs.	Diamonds
The book	vs.	The movie
Autograph	vs.	Photograph
CDs	vs.	Cassettes
Aretha	vs.	Mariah
Walking	vs.	Jogging
Giving	vs.	Receiving
Tailored	vs.	Casual
TV	vs.	Films

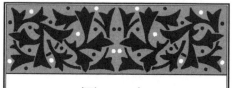

THAT'S
ENTERTAINMENT

Right now, my favorite:

    Music is _____

    Male singer is _____

    Female singer is _____

When I was a kid, my favorite:

    Music was _____

    Male singer was _____

    Female singer was _____

The hottest group right now is _____

My all-time favorite group/band is _____

The group that tops my chart now is _____

The last movie I saw was _____

    starring _____

    The rating I give this film is _____

My all-time favorite film is _____

My all-time favorite actor is _____

My current favorite actor is _____

My all-time favorite actress is _____

My current favorite actress is _____

The movie hunk who tops my list is _____

The glamour girl who's first with me is _____

I'd have to be dragged by my hair to see _____
_____ in a movie

The best show on TV today is _____

The TV show I'd never watch is _____

I wish they'd bring back this show _____

Reruns I never miss are _____

_____

The cartoon show I enjoy is _____

TV shows I watch on a regular basis are *(check off all that apply):*

     ❑ Evening news   ❑ Talk shows

     ❑ Soap operas   ❑ Quiz/Game shows

     ❑ Food shows   ❑ Political programs

     ❑ Live sports events   ❑ Weather stations

     ❑ Nature programs   ❑ Shopping shows

     ❑ Shock jocks   ❑ Sitcoms

     ❑ Dramatic series   ❑ Awards shows

     ❑ Movies   ❑ Detective/Police series

     ❑ Other _____

If I could be in a TV show it would be _____

    The character I would play is _____

My favorite childhood book was _____

The books I'd give my children to read are _____

_____

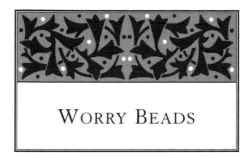

WORRY BEADS

Things that worry me are *(check all that apply):*

❏ Money ❏ Terrorism ❏ Abandonment ❏ Illness

❏ Failure ❏ Aging ❏ Weight gain ❏ Crime

❏ My family ❏ Flying ❏ Rejection ❏ Death

❏ War ❏ Driving ❏ Global warming ❏ Work/School

❏ Other _____

My biggest worry is _____

A natural catastrophe I most fear is _____

A natural disaster I experienced was _____

Something I worry might fail is _____

I worry about *(answer "usually," "sometimes," or "never"):*

Speaking in front of people _____

Trying on clothes in a dressing room _____

Not being taken seriously _____

Getting lost _____

Crowds _____

Being alone _____

Phone call in the middle of the night _____

Not being invited out _____

Driving at night _____

Driving in bad weather _____

Going home alone _____

Losing my job _____

My complexion _____

Being followed _____

Losing things _____

Breaking up with my loved one _____

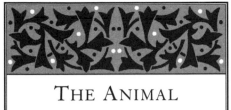

THE ANIMAL KINGDOM

I consider myself more ❑ a dog person ❑ a cat person

The animal I most fear is _____

An insect that really bugs me is _____

An animal that should be extinct is _____

My favorite dinosaur is _____

My favorite bird is _____

My feeling toward these animals is:

    Snakes _____

    Monkeys _____

    Elephants _____

    Kittens _____

    Puppies _____

    Horses _____

My current pets are _____

Past pets I've had are _____

The pet I miss most is _____

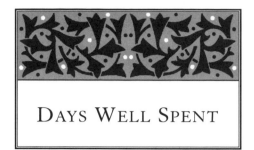

DAYS WELL SPENT

How I spend an average weekday *(list how much time you spend daily)*:

At work/school _____ hours _____ minutes

With the kids _____ hours _____ minutes

With friends _____ hours _____ minutes

Bathing/Grooming _____ hours _____ minutes

Exercising _____ hours _____ minutes

Doing household chores _____ hours _____ minutes

Talking on the phone _____ hours _____ minutes

Watching TV _____ hours _____ minutes

On the computer _____ hours _____ minutes

Eating and preparing meals _____ hours _____ minutes

Traveling _____ hours _____ minutes

Clubs/Organizations _____ hours _____ minutes

Hobbies _____ hours _____ minutes

Shopping _____ hours _____ minutes

Sleeping _____ hours _____ minutes

Other _____ _____ hours _____ minutes

My typical weekend is spent doing ____ _____

usually with _____

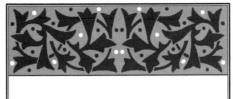

GLORIOUS FOOD

My favorite foods are:

_____

_____

_____

Foods that really turn me off are:

_____

_____

_____

The dish I most enjoy preparing is _____

    In brief, the recipe is:

    _____

    _____

    _____

The dish I make that everyone raves about is _____

I eat my meals at home   ❑ almost always   ❑ usually   ❑ not if I can help it

I like to barbecue   ❑ Yes   ❑ No   I like to attend barbecues   ❑ Yes   ❑ No

I send out for food   ❑ almost daily   ❑ weekly   ❑ monthly   ❑ hardly ever

When I send out I usually order from _____

and I usually order _____

My favorite restaurant is _____

located at _____

What I generally have is:

Cocktail/Beverage _____

Appetizer _____

Soup _____

Entrée/Main course _____

Side dishes _____

Dessert _____

The ethnic cuisine I'm most addicted to is _____

The fast food I often crave is _____

My favorite alcoholic drink is _____

My favorite nonalcoholic drink is _____

At lunchtime I can be found at _____

     having _____

My perfect meal would be *(fill in with your favorites):*

     Breakfast _____

     Lunch _____

     Dinner _____

     Dessert _____

When I watch TV or a movie I snack on _____

My favorite comfort food is _____

Childhood comfort foods that still work for me are _____

_____

The contents of my refrigerator right now: _____

_____

_____

During the past year I   ❏ have   ❏ have not been on a diet.

     The type of diet was _____

     It   ❏ was   ❏ was not successful because _____

_____

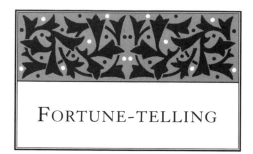

FORTUNE-TELLING

If I won the lottery, the first thing I'd do is _____

_____

The first luxury I'd buy is _____

The first place I'd go to is _____

A debt I would pay is _____

I'd share my good fortune with _____

The charity I'd give to is _____

The stock I would buy first is _____

A time I splurged on myself was _____

An inherited luxury I own is _____

My heart's desire:

Chauffeur and limo	❑ Definitely	❑ Not for me
Personal physician	❑ Definitely	❑ Not for me
Personal therapist	❑ Definitely	❑ Not for me
Personal astrologer	❑ Definitely	❑ Not for me
Live-in housekeeper	❑ Definitely	❑ Not for me
Nanny	❑ Definitely	❑ Not for me
Gardener	❑ Definitely	❑ Not for me
Pool and pool boy	❑ Definitely	❑ Not for me
Personal trainer	❑ Definitely	❑ Not for me
Personal hairdresser	❑ Definitely	❑ Not for me
Cook	❑ Definitely	❑ Not for me
Laundress	❑ Definitely	❑ Not for me
Butler	❑ Definitely	❑ Not for me
Private secretary	❑ Definitely	❑ Not for me
Seamstress	❑ Definitely	❑ Not for me
Personal shopper	❑ Definitely	❑ Not for me
Dietitian/Nutritionist	❑ Definitely	❑ Not for me
Manicurist	❑ Definitely	❑ Not for me
Makeup artist	❑ Definitely	❑ Not for me
Masseur/Masseuse	❑ Definitely	❑ Not for me
Decorator	❑ Definitely	❑ Not for me
Dog walker	❑ Definitely	❑ Not for me

The most expensive meal I ever ate was at _____

    The occasion was _____

The costliest gift I ever bought was _____

    I gave it to _____

The most expensive gift I received was _____

    Given to me by _____

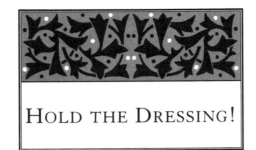

HOLD THE DRESSING!

My favorite clothing designer is _____

I most enjoy shopping for clothes at *(check all that apply):*

❑ Department stores   ❑ Boutiques

❑ Off-price stores/outlets   ❑ Thrift shops

❑ Mail-order catalogs   ❑ The Internet

❑ TV shopping clubs   ❑ Other _____

I could max out my credit card shopping at _____

The person I like to shop with is _____

I consider myself ❑ stylish ❑ nonconformist ❑ faddish ❑ uninterested

❑ other _____

The words I'd use to describe my personal style are:

_____

_____

The color I look best in is _____

The colors I usually wear are _____

The accessories I prefer are _____

_____

The last item of clothing I bought was _____

The most expensive item in my closet is _____

The most comfortable item I own is _____

I feel like a movie star when I wear my _____

To work/school, I usually wear _____

I could really use a new _____

Right now, I'm wearing _____

which I bought at _____

on _____

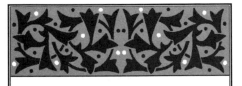

TOYS AND THINGS
(check the appropriate box)

Home	❑ Have it	❑ Want it	❑ Don't care
Vacation home	❑ Have it	❑ Want it	❑ Don't care
Condo/co-op apartment	❑ Have it	❑ Want it	❑ Don't care
Motor home	❑ Have it	❑ Want it	❑ Don't care
VCR	❑ Have it	❑ Want it	❑ Don't care
Large-screen TV	❑ Have it	❑ Want it	❑ Don't care
Mini TV	❑ Have it	❑ Want it	❑ Don't care
Satellite TV	❑ Have it	❑ Want it	❑ Don't care
Computer	❑ Have it	❑ Want it	❑ Don't care
Camera	❑ Have it	❑ Want it	❑ Don't care
Video camera	❑ Have it	❑ Want it	❑ Don't care
CD player	❑ Have it	❑ Want it	❑ Don't care

Sports equipment *(list):*

_____	❑ Have it	❑ Want it	❑ Don't care
_____	❑ Have it	❑ Want it	❑ Don't care
_____	❑ Have it	❑ Want it	❑ Don't care
Cell phone	❑ Have it	❑ Want it	❑ Don't care
Car	❑ Have it	❑ Want it	❑ Don't care

Second car	❑ Have it	❑ Want it	❑ Don't care
All-terrain vehicle	❑ Have it	❑ Want it	❑ Don't care
Recreational vehicle	❑ Have it	❑ Want it	❑ Don't care
Motorcycle	❑ Have it	❑ Want it	❑ Don't care

Jewelry *(list):*

_____	❑ Have it	❑ Want it	❑ Don't care
_____	❑ Have it	❑ Want it	❑ Don't care
_____	❑ Have it	❑ Want it	❑ Don't care
Designer wardrobe	❑ Have it	❑ Want it	❑ Don't care
Boat	❑ Have it	❑ Want it	❑ Don't care
Plane	❑ Have it	❑ Want it	❑ Don't care

Home appliance *(list):*

_____	❑ Have it	❑ Want it	❑ Don't care
_____	❑ Have it	❑ Want it	❑ Don't care
_____	❑ Have it	❑ Want it	❑ Don't care
Microwave oven	❑ Have it	❑ Want it	❑ Don't care
Good china	❑ Have it	❑ Want it	❑ Don't care
Good silverware	❑ Have it	❑ Want it	❑ Don't care
Expensive cookware	❑ Have it	❑ Want it	❑ Don't care

Other *(list):*

_____	❑ Have it	❑ Want it	❑ Don't care
_____	❑ Have it	❑ Want it	❑ Don't care

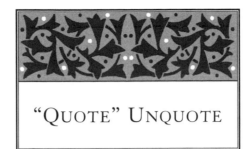

"Quote" Unquote

One can never be too rich or too thin ❑ Agree ❑ Disagree

It is better to have loved and lost
    than never to have loved at all ❑ Agree ❑ Disagree

Winning isn't everything—it's the only thing ❑ Agree ❑ Disagree

It doesn't matter what they say about me,
    as long as they spell my name right ❑ Agree ❑ Disagree

When I'm good I'm very, very good,
    but when I'm bad I'm better ❑ Agree ❑ Disagree

A friend is someone who knows all about you,
    but likes you anyway ❑ Agree ❑ Disagree

The best is yet to come ❑ Agree ❑ Disagree

Love is all there is ❑ Agree ❑ Disagree

A penny saved is a penny earned ❑ Agree ❑ Disagree

He who laughs last, laughs best ❑ Agree ❑ Disagree

He who laughs, lasts! ❑ Agree ❑ Disagree

Don't get mad, get even ❑ Agree ❑ Disagree

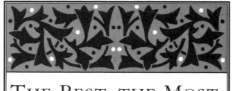

THE BEST, THE MOST, THE WORST

	In My Lifetime	*Of All Time*
World's most famous man	_____	_____
World's most famous woman	_____	_____
World's most evil despot	_____	_____
Greatest spiritual leader	_____	_____
The top inventions	_____	_____
	_____	_____
	_____	_____
The most useless invention	_____	_____
The top discoveries	_____	_____
	_____	_____
	_____	_____
Most feared disease	_____	_____
The top medical breakthrough	_____	_____

Best U.S. president _____ _____

Worst U.S. president _____ _____

Most powerful politician _____ _____

Most significant monarch _____ _____

Most infamous scandal _____ _____

Most notorious crime _____ _____

Worst disaster _____ _____

Most brilliant male thinker _____ _____

Most brilliant female thinker _____ _____

Dumbest public figure _____ _____

World's richest person _____ _____

Most handsome man _____ _____

Most beautiful woman _____ _____

Best baseball team _____ _____

Best football team _____ _____

Best basketball team _____ _____

World's greatest athlete   _____   _____

Best actor   _____   _____

Best actress   _____   _____

Best male entertainer   _____   _____

Best female entertainer   _____   _____

Most important fashion   _____   _____

Most important document   _____   _____

Most significant law   _____   _____

Greatest natural wonder   _____   _____

Greatest natural calamity   _____   _____

Greatest man-made structure   _____   _____

Man's most useless structure   _____   _____

Best composer   _____   _____

Best artist   _____   _____

Best author   _____   _____

Most celebrated love affair   _____   _____

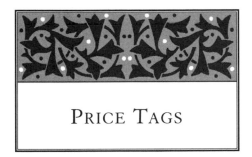

PRICE TAGS

(if you don't know the exact amount, use an average)

Today's date:_____

Daily newspaper	$ _____
Video rental	$ _____
Bag of popcorn	$ _____
Box of breakfast cereal	$ _____
Pair of sneakers	$ _____
CD	$ _____
Gallon of regular gas	$ _____
Gallon of premium gas	$ _____
Movie theater ticket	$ _____
Dinner at my favorite restaurant	$ _____
Meal at a fast-food restaurant	$ _____
Hardcover book	$ _____
Dozen roses	$ _____
Local outside telephone call	$ _____
Quart of orange juice	$ _____
New economy car	$ _____
New luxury car	$ _____
Quart of milk	$ _____
Order-out pizza	$ _____
Tube of toothpaste	$ _____
Six-pack of beer	$ _____
T-shirt	$ _____
Pair of jeans	$ _____
Average dress	$ _____

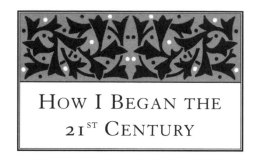

HOW I BEGAN THE 21ST CENTURY

N E W   Y E A R ' S   E V E

I made my plans/reservations for New Year's Eve on _____

I started my celebrations at _____ P.M. The weather was _____

To ring in the 21st century, I was at _____
_____

I was accompanied by _____

Other people there were _____
_____

My New Year's Eve outfit was _____
_____
_____

I bought it at _____ on _____ and it cost $_____

I looked   ❑ fabulous   ❑ very good   ❑ so-so   ❑ it wasn't the real me   ❑ ugh!

The best-dressed person there was _____

who wore _____

The worst-dressed person there was _____

who wore _____

My last meal of the 20th century consisted of _____

_____

The food was ❏ extraordinary ❏ okay ❏ what you'd expect ❏ pretty bad

I drank _____

which was ❏ far too much ❏ not enough ❏ just the right amount

At the stroke of midnight, I was at _____

with _____

I kissed _____

_____

and I thought _____

_____

Other ways I celebrated the new millennium at midnight were _____

_____

My top resolution for the new millennium was _____

_____

My other resolutions were _____

_____

_____

The resolution I most want to keep is _____

The resolution I need to keep is _____

The resolution I'm most likely to keep is _____

I make New Year's resolutions ❏ always ❏ usually ❏ occasionally ❏ never

I keep most resolutions I make ❏ always ❏ usually ❏ occasionally ❏ never

A resolution I make every year is _____

A resolution I break every year is _____

Resolutions I would like others to make are:

Name   *Resolution*

_____   _____

_____   _____

_____   _____

_____   _____

New Year's Eve highlights were _____

_____

The main subjects discussed were _____

_____

The music I heard was _____

What made this New Year's Eve most memorable was _____

_____

because _____

What I'd most like to forget about the night is _____

_____

because _____

The most unusual/interesting thing that happened was _____

_____

    because_____

I thought New Year's Eve was   ❏ magical   ❏ ordinary   ❏ boring   ❏ a dud!

    because_____

_____

If I could have spent the night anywhere else it would have been at _____

_____

    because _____

If I could have spent the night with anyone else it would have been _____

_____

    because _____

The total cost of the evening was $ _____

I went to sleep at _____ feeling/thinking_____

_____

_____

_____

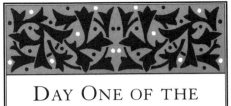

DAY ONE OF THE NEW MILLENNIUM

On the first day of the new millennium, I woke up at _____

and the weather was _____

The first thing I felt/thought about was _____

_____

The first thing I did was _____

_____

The first person I spoke to was _____

and we discussed _____

_____

I spent most of the day at _____

_____

doing _____

_____

The best thing that happened to me was _____

_____

The worst thing that happened to me was _____

_____

The top news of the day is _____

_____

The results of the predicted Y2K problem are _____

_____

Other predictions for the new millennium were _____

_____

and the results are _____

_____

At the end of the 20th century, the Dow closed at _____

The biggest problems facing the world in the new millennium are:

_____

_____

My personal goals for the new millennium are *(list in order of importance):*

_____

_____

_____

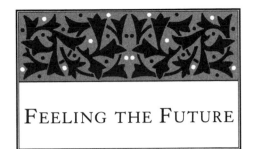

FEELING THE FUTURE

The worst things about growing old will be _____

_____

_____

What will make me feel most secure in the future is _____

_____

_____

Living for the moment is _____

_____

Regretting the past is _____

_____

Playing it safe is _____

_____

Going for broke is _____

_____

The things I wish would not change are:

_____

_____

_____

How I feel about the future *(write your innermost thoughts):*

_____

_____

_____

_____

_____

_____

_____

_____

_____

_____

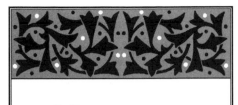

I Predict . . .

In the years to come:

My marital status will be _____

My body shape will be _____

My general health will be _____

My social life will become _____

A new activity I will take up is _____

An activity I will drop is _____

The climate where I live will become _____

I will relocate to another city/town   ❑ Yes ❑ No

I will get a new pet   ❑ Yes ❑ No

I will redecorate my home   ❏ Yes ❏ No

I will have a new job   ❏ Yes ❏ No

I will change my political affiliation   ❏ Yes ❏ No

On the financial front, I will be   ❏ better off ❏ worse off ❏ about the same

The stock market will   ❏ go through the roof ❏ stay the same ❏ take a dive

The next U.S. president will be _____

There will be a female president soon   ❏ Agree   ❏ Disagree

There will be a nonwhite president soon   ❏ Agree   ❏ Disagree

Euthanasia will be permitted   ❏ Agree   ❏ Disagree

Abortion will continue to be legal   ❏ Agree   ❏ Disagree

Overpopulation will endanger the world   ❏ Agree   ❏ Disagree

The draft will be reinstituted   ❏ Agree   ❏ Disagree

Homosexual marriages will be accepted   ❏ Agree   ❏ Disagree

Marijuana will be legalized   ❏ Agree   ❏ Disagree

Biological warfare will be our prime fear   ❏ Agree   ❏ Disagree

There will be a four-day work week   ❏ Agree   ❏ Disagree

Global warming will be a real danger   ❏ Agree   ❏ Disagree

Science will enable men to become pregnant   ❏ Agree   ❏ Disagree

Cloning humans will be common practice   ❏ Agree   ❏ Disagree

Artificial organs will be common   ❏ Agree   ❏ Disagree

There will be a cure for cancer   ❏ Agree   ❏ Disagree

Pills will replace food   ❏ Agree   ❏ Disagree

Holidays will include travel to other planets   ❑ Agree   ❑ Disagree

Except for zoos, wild animals will be extinct   ❑ Agree   ❑ Disagree

The world will   ❑ enjoy lasting peace   ❑ face Armageddon   ❑ see few changes

The environment will   ❑ improve greatly   ❑ collapse   ❑ remain about the same

People will live to be an average of _____ years old

I foresee these medical breakthroughs:

_____

_____

_____

We are in a new century and a new millennium. After giving it some consideration, my top predictions for what the future will bring are:

_____

_____

_____

_____

_____

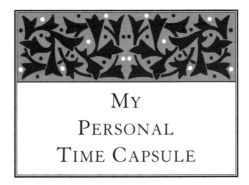

My
Personal
Time Capsule

What I would include in my time capsule for the new millennium:

*To be opened in the year*_____ *by* _____

_____

_____

_____

_____

_____

_____

_____

_____

_____

_____

_____

_____

_____